INTRODUCTION

The human diet has been a topic of debate for centuries, with different schools of thought and beliefs guiding what we eat and how we live. From vegetarianism and veganism to the paleo diet and keto diet, there is no shortage of dietary patterns and approaches to achieving optimal health and well-being.

One such dietary pattern that has gained traction in recent years is the carnivorous diet, which advocates for a diet consisting primarily of animal-based products. While this diet may seem extreme and controversial to some, it has garnered a loyal following of individuals who have reported significant health benefits from adopting this way of eating.

But what exactly is the carnivorous diet, and what makes it so unique? In this book, we will explore the ins and outs of the carnivorous diet, from its historical roots to the latest research on its potential benefits and risks.

We will delve into the science behind the carnivorous diet, including the role of protein and fat in the diet and how the body processes nutrients. We will also examine the impact of the carnivorous diet on weight loss, improved blood markers, and increased energy, as well as the ethical and environmental considerations that come with consuming animal-based products.

Additionally, we will provide practical advice on how to implement a carnivorous diet, including common pitfalls to avoid and tips for staying on track. We will also address concerns around nutrient deficiencies and health risks and provide strategies for mitigating these risks.

Whether you're a curious observer or a committed carnivore, this book will provide you with the knowledge and tools to make informed decisions about your health and dietary choices. So let's dive into the world of the carnivorous diet and discover what this way of eating has to offer.

CHAPTER ONE

Introduction

Explanation Of The Carnivorous Diet

The carnivorous diet, also known as a zero-carb or all-meat diet, is a way of eating that focuses exclusively on animal-based foods, such as meat, fish, eggs, and dairy products. The diet typically excludes all plant-based foods, including fruits, vegetables, grains, and legumes.

The primary macronutrients in the carnivorous diet are protein and fat. Animal-based foods are rich in high-quality protein and healthy fats, including omega-3 fatty acids and conjugated linoleic acid (CLA), which have been linked to a wide range of health benefits.

Proponents of the carnivorous diet argue that it is more natural for humans to eat a diet primarily composed of animal-based foods, as our early ancestors did. They also suggest that the diet can help with a variety of health issues, including weight loss, improved blood markers, and increased energy levels.

However, critics of the carnivorous diet argue that it is not a balanced or sustainable way of eating in the long term. They suggest that the diet may be lacking in certain nutrients, such as fiber, vitamins, and minerals, which are typically found in plant-based foods. They also argue that the high intake of saturated fat and cholesterol in the diet may increase the risk of heart disease and other chronic illnesses.

Overall, the carnivorous diet remains a controversial way of eating, with both potential benefits and risks. It is important to consult with a healthcare professional before making any significant changes to your diet.

Brief history of the diet

The carnivorous diet, as a way of eating, has a long and complex history that spans back to the earliest days of human civilization. While there is no one definitive origin story for the diet, there are a number of key cultural and historical factors that have contributed to its development over time.

One of the earliest examples of a carnivorous diet can be found in the diets of our ancient ancestors, who relied heavily on animal-based foods for their sustenance. Early humans were hunter-gatherers who relied on hunting wild animals and fishing in order to obtain the protein and fat necessary for survival. This diet continued for thousands of years, until the advent of agriculture around 10,000 years ago.

With the rise of agriculture, humans began to shift towards a more plant-based diet, with grains, fruits, and vegetables becoming staple foods in many cultures. However, the consumption of animal-based foods continued to play an important role in many societies, particularly those that relied on livestock for their livelihood.

One notable example of a carnivorous diet can be found in the traditional diets of many indigenous cultures, particularly those of the Arctic regions. These cultures relied heavily on animal-based foods, such as whale blubber, seal meat, and fish, for their sustenance. The Inuit people, for example, have been noted for their high consumption of animal-based foods and their relatively low incidence of chronic disease.

In more recent history, the carnivorous diet has been associated with various cultural movements and health fads. The Atkins diet, which gained popularity in the 1990s, emphasized the consumption of high-protein, low-carbohydrate foods, including meat, fish, and eggs. The Paleo diet, which became popular in the early 2000s, emphasizes the consumption of foods that were available to our early ancestors, including meat, fish, nuts, and seeds.

More recently, the carnivorous diet has gained a following among certain health and fitness enthusiasts, who believe that the diet can help with weight loss, improved energy levels, and other health benefits. However, the diet remains controversial, with many experts warning of potential risks associated with a high intake of animal-based foods, such as increased risk of heart disease and other chronic illnesses.

Overall, the history of the carnivorous diet reflects the

complex interplay between cultural traditions, scientific knowledge, and individual preferences and beliefs. While the diet remains a controversial and debated topic, it continues to attract interest and attention from those who seek to optimize their health and well-being through their dietary choices.

CHAPTER TWO

The Science of the Carnivorous Diet

Explanation Of How The Body Processes Nutrients

The human body relies on a complex system of processes to break down and utilize the nutrients found in food. These processes begin in the mouth and continue throughout the digestive system, with different enzymes and hormones working together to extract the energy and nutrients needed to fuel the body's various functions.

Digestion begins in the mouth, where food is chewed and mixed with saliva. Saliva contains enzymes that begin to break down carbohydrates and fats, while also moistening and lubricating the food to make it easier to swallow.

Once the food has been swallowed, it travels down the esophagus and into the stomach. Here, it is mixed with stomach acid and digestive enzymes, which continue to break down the food and kill any harmful bacteria or viruses that may be present. The stomach also plays an important role in regulating the rate at which food is released into the small intestine, where most of the nutrient absorption occurs.

In the small intestine, the food is further broken down by enzymes produced by the pancreas and small intestine itself. Carbohydrates are broken down into simple sugars, proteins are broken down into amino acids, and fats are broken down into fatty acids and glycerol. These nutrients are then absorbed into the bloodstream and transported to various tissues and organs throughout the body.

The process of nutrient absorption is facilitated by the villi and microvilli, which are tiny finger-like projections that line the walls of the small intestine. These structures increase the surface area of the intestine, allowing for greater absorption of nutrients into the bloodstream.

Once the nutrients have been absorbed, they are

transported to the liver for processing. The liver plays a key role in regulating the levels of nutrients and hormones in the bloodstream, while also helping to remove toxins and waste products from the body.

Carbohydrates are converted into glucose, which can be used immediately by the body for energy or stored in the liver and muscles as glycogen for later use. Excess glucose is converted into fat and stored in adipose tissue.

Proteins are broken down into amino acids, which are used to build and repair tissues throughout the body. Any excess amino acids are converted into glucose or fat and stored in the body.

Fats are broken down into fatty acids and glycerol, which can be used for energy or stored in adipose tissue for later use. The liver also plays a key role in the synthesis of certain types of fats, including cholesterol and triglycerides.

In addition to the macronutrients, the body also requires a variety of micronutrients, such as vitamins and minerals, in order to maintain optimal health and function. These nutrients are typically obtained through the diet, with the body using various mechanisms to regulate their absorption and utilization.

Vitamins and minerals are absorbed in the small intestine along with other nutrients, with the body using specialized transporters and binding proteins to ensure that they are delivered to the tissues and organs that need them most. Many vitamins and minerals also play important roles in enzymatic reactions and other physiological processes throughout the body, helping to support overall health and well-being.

Overall, the process of nutrient digestion and absorption is a complex and highly regulated system that plays a critical role in supporting optimal health and function. By understanding how the body processes nutrients, individuals can make informed choices about their dietary habits, ensuring that they are getting the nutrients they need to support their overall health and well-being.

Comparison Of Nutrient Profiles Between Animal-Based And Plant-Based Foods

The nutrient profiles of animal-based and plant-based

foods differ in several ways. While both types of foods contain essential nutrients, the specific types and amounts of nutrients present can vary significantly. Here, we will compare the nutrient profiles of animal-based and plant-based foods across several key categories.

- Protein: Animal-based foods tend to be higher in protein than plant-based foods. This is because animal-based foods, such as meat, fish, and dairy, contain all of the essential amino acids, whereas most plant-based foods are lacking in one or more essential amino acids. However, plant-based protein sources such as legumes, nuts, and whole grains can be combined to provide all of the essential amino acids, making them a good option for vegetarians and vegans.
- Fats: Animal-based foods tend to be higher in saturated fats, while plant-based foods are higher in unsaturated fats. Saturated fats are associated with an increased risk of heart disease, while unsaturated fats can help reduce the risk of heart disease and other chronic illnesses.
- Omega-3 Fatty Acids: Animal-based sources of omega-3 fatty acids, such as fatty fish, are considered the most bioavailable and beneficial sources of this essential nutrient. However, plant-based sources of omega-3s, such as flaxseeds, chia seeds, and walnuts, can also provide significant amounts of this nutrient.
- Vitamins and Minerals: Plant-based foods tend to be higher in vitamins and minerals, such as

vitamin C, vitamin A, folate, and potassium, while animal-based foods are higher in vitamins and minerals such as vitamin B12, iron, and zinc. Vitamin B12 is only found in animal-based foods, making it a key nutrient for vegetarians and vegans to supplement.

- Fiber: Plant-based foods tend to be higher in dietary fiber, which is important for promoting digestive health and reducing the risk of chronic diseases such as heart disease, diabetes, and certain types of cancer.
- Phytonutrients: Plant-based foods are also rich in phytonutrients, which are compounds that provide various health benefits. These include antioxidants, which help protect against oxidative damage and inflammation, and phytochemicals, which can help reduce the risk of chronic diseases such as cancer and heart disease.

Overall, both animal-based and plant-based foods can provide essential nutrients and support optimal health and well-being. However, the nutrient profiles of these foods can vary significantly, making it important to consume a variety of foods from both sources in order to ensure a well-rounded and balanced diet.

It is worth noting that some studies have suggested that plant-based diets may be associated with certain health benefits, such as reduced risk of heart disease and lower blood pressure. However, other studies have found conflicting results, and it is important to note that individual factors such as genetics, lifestyle, and overall dietary patterns can also play a role in determining the health benefits of a particular diet.

Ultimately, the best approach is to focus on consuming a variety of whole foods from both animal and plant sources, while limiting processed and refined foods. This can help ensure a balanced and nutrient-rich diet that supports optimal health and well-being.

The Role Of Protein And Fat In The Diet

Protein and fat are two of the three macronutrients essential to the human diet, with the third being carbohydrates. They each play important roles in supporting the body's functions and maintaining optimal health. Here, we will delve into the specific roles of protein and fat in the diet.

- Protein: Protein is a crucial component of all cells in the body, and it is needed to build and repair tissues, produce enzymes and hormones, and support the immune system. It is made up of amino acids, which are the building blocks of protein. There are nine essential amino acids that the body cannot produce on its own and must obtain from food sources. Protein is particularly important for building and repairing muscle tissue, making it a key nutrient for athletes and individuals engaging in regular physical activity. Additionally, protein can help promote feelings of satiety, or fullness, making it a useful nutrient for weight management. Sources of protein include animal-based foods such as meat, poultry, fish, eggs, and dairy, as well as plant-based sources such as legumes, nuts, seeds, and whole grains. Animal-based sources of protein tend to be more complete, meaning they contain all nine essential amino acids in the right proportions, while plant-based sources may need to be combined to provide all essential amino acids.

- Fat: Fat is an essential nutrient that plays several important roles in the body, including providing energy, supporting the absorption of fat-soluble vitamins, and maintaining healthy skin and hair. It also serves as an important structural component of cell membranes. There are three main types of dietary fat: saturated, unsaturated, and trans. Saturated fat is found primarily in animal-based foods such as meat and dairy, while unsaturated fat is found in plant-based foods such as nuts, seeds, and vegetable oils. Trans fats are typically found in processed foods and should be avoided as they have been linked to increased risk of heart disease. Unsaturated fats, particularly omega-3 fatty acids found in fatty fish, have been linked to various health benefits, including reducing inflammation and improving brain function. However, it is important to consume fats in moderation, as they are calorie-dense and can contribute to weight gain if consumed in excess.

Overall, both protein and fat play important roles in the human diet, and consuming a balanced diet that includes a variety of protein and fat sources is key to supporting optimal health and well-being. It is recommended that adults consume at least 0.8 grams of protein per kilogram of body weight per day, with individual needs varying based on factors such as age, sex, and activity level. Fat should make up around 20-35% of total daily calorie intake, with a focus on consuming unsaturated fats from plant-based sources.

The Impact Of The Carnivorous Diet On The Body, Including Weight Loss, Improved Blood Markers, And Increased Energy

The carnivorous diet, also known as the all-meat diet, is a diet that primarily consists of animal-based foods such as meat, poultry, fish, and eggs. While the diet is controversial and not widely accepted by mainstream health organizations, some individuals report significant benefits from following a carnivorous diet. Here, we will discuss the impact of the carnivorous diet on the body, including potential benefits such as weight loss, improved blood markers, and increased energy.

- Weight Loss: One of the most commonly reported benefits of the carnivorous diet is weight loss. This is likely due to the high protein content of the diet, which can help promote feelings of fullness and reduce overall calorie intake. Additionally, the elimination of processed and high-carbohydrate foods that are common in the standard Western diet may also contribute to weight loss. In one study, overweight and obese individuals who followed a low-carbohydrate, high-protein diet for six months lost more weight and body fat compared to those who followed a low-fat diet. Another study found that a high-protein diet resulted in greater fat loss and preservation of muscle mass compared to a low-protein diet. However, it is important to note that weight loss on the carnivorous diet may not be sustainable in the long term, and the high intake of saturated fat and cholesterol from animal-based foods may increase the risk of heart disease.
- Improved Blood Markers: The carnivorous diet has been shown to have a positive impact on several blood markers, including cholesterol levels, blood pressure, and blood sugar control. Several studies

have shown that a low-carbohydrate, high-protein diet can improve cholesterol levels by increasing levels of "good" HDL cholesterol and decreasing levels of "bad" LDL cholesterol. Additionally, a high-protein diet may help improve blood sugar control and insulin sensitivity, which can be beneficial for individuals with type 2 diabetes. Another potential benefit of the carnivorous diet is improved blood pressure control. A study of individuals with high blood pressure found that a high-protein diet led to greater reductions in blood pressure compared to a low-protein diet.

- Increased Energy: Some individuals report increased energy and improved mental clarity when following a carnivorous diet. This may be due to the elimination of processed and high-carbohydrate foods that can cause energy crashes and brain fog. Additionally, the high protein content of the carnivorous diet may provide a sustained source of energy throughout the day. Protein is also essential for building and repairing muscle tissue, which can contribute to overall physical performance and energy levels. However, it is important to note that the carnivorous diet may not be suitable for everyone, and some individuals may experience negative side effects such as constipation, fatigue, and nutrient deficiencies. It is important to work with a healthcare provider to ensure that all nutrient needs are being met while following a carnivorous diet.

In conclusion, while the carnivorous diet is not widely

accepted by mainstream health organizations and there is limited research on its long-term effects, some individuals report significant benefits from following the diet. These potential benefits include weight loss, improved blood markers, and increased energy. However, it is important to carefully consider the potential risks and side effects of the diet and work with a healthcare provider to ensure that all nutrient needs are being met.

CHAPTER THREE

The Philosophy of the

Carnivorous Diet

The Ethical Considerations Of A Carnivorous Diet

The decision to follow a carnivorous diet is not only a personal health choice but also an ethical one. The ethics surrounding the consumption of animal products have been debated for many years, and the carnivorous diet has been criticized for its potential negative impact on animal welfare and the environment. Here, we will discuss the ethical considerations of a carnivorous diet.

- Animal Welfare: One of the main ethical concerns with the carnivorous diet is the treatment of animals. The meat industry is known for its poor treatment of animals, including overcrowding, limited access to food and water, and the use of hormones and antibiotics. Many people believe that consuming animal products perpetuates this cruel treatment of animals and that it is unethical to support an industry that prioritizes profit over the welfare of living beings. The carnivorous diet also requires the consumption of a large amount of animal products, which can lead to an increased demand for meat and other animal-based foods. This increased demand can lead to the further exploitation and mistreatment of animals.

- Environmental Impact: Another ethical concern of the carnivorous diet is its impact on the environment. The meat industry is a significant contributor to greenhouse gas emissions, deforestation, and water pollution. The production of animal products requires large amounts of land, water, and energy, and the waste produced by the industry can lead to environmental degradation. The carnivorous diet also requires the consumption of a large amount of animal products, which can contribute to the environmental impact of the meat industry. Additionally, the elimination of plant-based foods from the diet can result in a limited variety of foods and a reliance on monoculture farming, which can lead to soil depletion and environmental damage.

- Alternative Approaches: While the ethical considerations of the carnivorous diet are significant, there are alternative approaches to consuming animal products that prioritize animal welfare and environmental sustainability.

These approaches include ethical and sustainable farming practices, such as grass-fed and free-range animal products, as well as plant-based diets that incorporate small amounts of animal products. Some people also choose to follow a nose-to-tail approach to the carnivorous diet, which involves consuming all parts of the animal, including organ meats and bones. This approach can reduce waste and honor the animal by utilizing all of its parts. Additionally, the use of alternative protein sources, such as plant-based protein powders and insect-based protein, can reduce the reliance on animal products and decrease the environmental impact of the diet.

- Personal Ethics: Ultimately, the decision to follow a carnivorous diet is a personal one that should consider individual ethical values and beliefs. Some individuals may prioritize personal health benefits over animal welfare and environmental concerns, while others may prioritize ethical and sustainable practices over personal health benefits. It is important to note that the ethics surrounding the consumption of animal products are complex and multifaceted, and there is no one-size-fits-all solution. However, individuals can make informed and ethical choices by researching and understanding the impact of their dietary choices on animal welfare, the environment, and personal health.

In conclusion, the ethical considerations of the carnivorous diet are significant and should be carefully considered when making dietary choices. The meat industry's poor treatment of animals and environmental impact are major ethical concerns, and alternative approaches to consuming animal products should be considered. Ultimately, individuals should make informed and ethical choices that align with their personal values and beliefs.

The Environmental Impact Of Meat Consumption

Meat consumption has a significant impact on the environment, contributing to various environmental issues such as deforestation, greenhouse gas emissions, water scarcity, and water pollution. In this article, we will explore the environmental impact of meat consumption in detail.

- Greenhouse Gas Emissions: The production of meat and other animal-based products is a significant contributor to greenhouse gas emissions. The livestock sector is responsible for approximately 14.5% of global greenhouse gas emissions, which is more than the emissions from the transportation sector. The primary greenhouse gas emitted by the livestock sector is methane, which is produced during enteric fermentation (digestion) in ruminant animals such as cattle, sheep, and goats. Methane has a much higher global warming potential than carbon dioxide and contributes to climate change. In addition to methane, the production of meat and animal-based products also generates carbon dioxide emissions from the energy used to produce feed and transport animals, as well as from deforestation for pasture and feed production.

- Deforestation: The production of meat and animal-based products is also a major driver of deforestation. Forests are often cleared to make way for pastureland, soybean fields, and other crops used for animal feed production. Deforestation not only contributes to greenhouse gas emissions but also leads to habitat destruction and biodiversity loss. The Amazon rainforest, for example, has been extensively cleared for cattle ranching, leading to the destruction of vital ecosystems and threatening the survival of numerous plant and animal species.

- Water Scarcity and Water Pollution: Meat production is also a significant contributor to water scarcity and water pollution. The livestock sector is responsible for approximately 8% of global freshwater use, and water consumption for animal production is expected to increase in the coming years. In addition to water consumption, the livestock sector is also a major source of water pollution. Animal waste and fertilizers used in feed production can contaminate waterways, leading to eutrophication and harmful algal blooms.

- Overfishing: The consumption of fish and seafood also has a significant impact on the environment. Overfishing and destructive fishing practices, such as bottom trawling, can lead to the depletion of fish stocks and damage to marine ecosystems. The use of fishing gear, such as longlines and gillnets, can also result in bycatch, the unintentional capture of non-target species. Bycatch can result in the death of non-target species, including endangered species such as sea turtles and sharks.

- Alternative Approaches: Reducing meat consumption and shifting towards plant-based diets is one approach to reducing the environmental impact of meat consumption. Plant-based diets require less land, water, and energy to produce and emit fewer greenhouse gas emissions than meat-based diets. Additionally, choosing sustainably sourced animal products can also help reduce the environmental impact of meat consumption. Grass-fed beef, for example, requires less energy and produces fewer greenhouse gas emissions than conventionally raised beef. Other approaches to reducing the environmental impact of meat consumption include reducing food waste, choosing products with minimal packaging, and supporting sustainable and responsible fishing practices.

The environmental impact of meat consumption is significant and should be carefully considered when making dietary choices. Meat production contributes to greenhouse gas emissions, deforestation, water scarcity, water pollution, and overfishing. Reducing meat consumption and shifting towards plant-based diets and sustainably sourced animal products can help reduce the environmental impact of meat consumption. By making informed and sustainable choices, we can work towards a more sustainable and environmentally responsible food system.

The Role Of Ancestral Diets In Informing The Carnivorous Diet

The carnivorous diet is based on the premise that humans evolved as apex predators, consuming primarily animal-based foods for millions of years. Proponents of the carnivorous diet argue that this ancestral diet is more in line with our genetic makeup and may offer numerous health benefits.

- Ancestral Diets: Ancestral diets, also known as

paleolithic or hunter-gatherer diets, refer to the dietary patterns of human ancestors before the advent of agriculture. These diets were based on the foods that were available in the natural environment and varied depending on geographic location and seasonality. Ancestral diets typically consisted of animal-based foods such as meat, fish, and eggs, as well as nuts, seeds, fruits, and vegetables. These foods were consumed in their whole, unprocessed form and did not include grains, dairy products, or processed foods. The theory behind the ancestral diet is that humans evolved to consume foods that were available in the natural environment, and that these foods provided optimal nutrition for our genetic makeup. Proponents of the ancestral diet argue that modern dietary patterns, which are high in processed foods and grains, are not in line with our genetic makeup and may contribute to numerous health problems.

- Role of Ancestral Diets in Informing the Carnivorous Diet: The carnivorous diet is based on the premise that humans evolved as apex predators, consuming primarily animal-based foods for millions of years. This dietary pattern is consistent with the dietary patterns of many ancestral cultures, which relied heavily on animal-based foods. Proponents of the carnivorous diet argue that animal-based foods provide optimal nutrition for human health and that many of the health problems associated with modern dietary patterns are the result of consuming too many processed foods and grains.

Research suggests that animal-based foods are a rich source of nutrients, including protein, vitamins, and minerals, that are essential for human health. These nutrients are often more bioavailable in animal-based foods than in plant-based foods, which may make them more effective in promoting optimal health. In addition to the nutrient content of animal-based foods, proponents of the carnivorous diet argue that animal-based foods may offer numerous health benefits that are not found in plant-based foods. For example, animal-based foods are a rich source of essential amino acids, which are important for muscle growth and repair. Animal-based foods also contain numerous micronutrients, such as iron, zinc, and vitamin B12, that are essential for optimal health.

- Impact on Human Health: While the carnivorous diet may offer numerous health benefits, it is important to note that this dietary pattern is not without controversy. Critics of the carnivorous diet argue that it may increase the risk of certain health problems, such as heart disease, due to its high saturated fat content. Research on the impact of the carnivorous diet on human health is limited, and more research is needed to fully understand the potential benefits and risks of this dietary pattern. However, some studies suggest that the carnivorous diet may offer numerous health benefits, including weight loss, improved blood sugar control, and improved markers of cardiovascular health.

The carnivorous diet is based on the premise that humans evolved as apex predators, consuming primarily animal-based foods for millions of years. Proponents of the carnivorous diet argue that this dietary pattern is more in line with our genetic makeup and may offer numerous health benefits.

Ancestral diets, such as paleolithic or hunter-gatherer diets, may offer insights into the dietary patterns of our ancestors and may inform the carnivorous diet. Research suggests that animal-based foods are a rich source of nutrients that are essential for human health, and that many of the health problems associated with modern dietary patterns may be the result of consuming too many processed foods and grains.

Iv. The Practical Application Of The Carnivorous Diet

How to implement a carnivorous diet

Implementing a carnivorous diet can be a significant dietary shift for some individuals, and it is important to approach this dietary pattern in a safe and sustainable manner. Here are some tips for implementing a carnivorous diet:

- Consult with a healthcare professional: Before starting any new dietary pattern, it is important to consult with a healthcare professional to ensure that it is safe and appropriate for your individual health needs. A healthcare professional can help you create a personalized dietary plan that meets your nutritional needs and supports optimal health.
- Choose high-quality animal-based foods: When following a carnivorous diet, it is important to choose high-quality animal-based foods that are nutrient-dense and minimally processed. Choose grass-fed beef, pasture-raised poultry and eggs, and wild-caught fish to ensure that you are getting the highest quality nutrition from your food.
- Include a variety of animal-based foods: While a carnivorous diet is primarily based on animal-based foods, it is important to include a variety of different types of animal-based foods to ensure that you are getting a wide range of nutrients. Incorporate beef, poultry, fish, eggs, and organ meats into your diet to ensure that you are getting a range of protein, vitamins, and minerals.
- Consider adding dairy products: While some individuals following a carnivorous diet choose to exclude dairy products, others may choose to include high-quality dairy products such as full-

fat cheese, yogurt, and cream. Dairy products are a rich source of calcium and other important nutrients, and can be a valuable addition to a carnivorous diet.

- Be mindful of your fat intake: Animal-based foods are typically high in fat, and it is important to be mindful of your fat intake when following a carnivorous diet. Choose lean cuts of meat, trim excess fat, and incorporate heart-healthy fats such as olive oil, avocado, and nuts to ensure that you are getting the right balance of fats in your diet.

- Incorporate low-carbohydrate vegetables: While a carnivorous diet is primarily based on animal-based foods, it is important to incorporate some low-carbohydrate vegetables into your diet to ensure that you are getting fiber and other important nutrients. Consider incorporating leafy greens, cruciferous vegetables, and other low-carbohydrate vegetables into your meals to ensure that you are getting a well-rounded and nutritious diet.

- Stay hydrated: Drinking plenty of water is important for overall health, and it is especially important when following a carnivorous diet. Animal-based foods tend to be high in protein, which can be dehydrating. Make sure to drink plenty of water throughout the day to stay hydrated and support optimal health.

- Monitor your nutrient intake: When following a carnivorous diet, it is important to monitor your nutrient intake to ensure that you are getting all of the essential nutrients that your body needs. Consider working with a healthcare professional

> or registered dietitian to track your nutrient intake and make adjustments as needed.
> - Listen to your body: As with any dietary pattern, it is important to listen to your body and make adjustments as needed. Pay attention to how you feel after eating certain foods, and make adjustments to your diet as needed to support optimal health and well-being.

In conclusion, implementing a carnivorous diet can be a significant dietary shift, but it can also offer numerous health benefits for some individuals. By choosing high-quality animal-based foods, incorporating a variety of animal-based foods, and being mindful of your fat intake and nutrient intake, you can safely and effectively implement a carnivorous diet that supports optimal health and well-being. As with any dietary pattern, it is important to consult with a healthcare professional and listen to your body to ensure that you are getting the right nutrition for your individual needs.

Common Pitfalls To Avoid

While a carnivorous diet can offer numerous health benefits for some individuals, there are also some common pitfalls to avoid when implementing this dietary pattern. Here are some common pitfalls to be aware of and tips for avoiding them:

- Not getting enough variety in your diet: While a carnivorous diet is primarily based on animal-based foods, it is important to get a variety of different types of animal-based foods to ensure that you are getting a wide range of nutrients. Incorporate beef, poultry, fish, eggs, and organ meats into your diet to ensure that you are getting a range of protein, vitamins, and minerals.
- Not getting enough fiber: Animal-based foods tend to be low in fiber, and it can be easy to fall short on this important nutrient when following a carnivorous diet. Consider incorporating low-carbohydrate vegetables such as leafy greens, cruciferous vegetables, and other non-starchy vegetables into your diet to ensure that you are getting enough fiber.
- Not monitoring your nutrient intake: When following a carnivorous diet, it is important to monitor your nutrient intake to ensure that you are getting all of the essential nutrients that your body needs. Consider working with a healthcare professional or registered dietitian to track your nutrient intake and make adjustments as needed.
- Overeating: While a carnivorous diet can be an effective way to support weight loss, it is important to be mindful of your portion sizes and avoid overeating. Choose high-quality, nutrient-dense foods and eat until you are satisfied, but not

overly full.

- Eating too much protein: While protein is an important nutrient, it is possible to consume too much protein when following a carnivorous diet. Aim to consume a moderate amount of protein, and be mindful of your fat intake to ensure that you are getting the right balance of macronutrients.
- Not getting enough hydration: Animal-based foods tend to be high in protein, which can be dehydrating. Make sure to drink plenty of water throughout the day to stay hydrated and support optimal health.
- Ignoring pre-existing medical conditions: Before starting any new dietary pattern, it is important to consult with a healthcare professional to ensure that it is safe and appropriate for your individual health needs. If you have pre-existing medical conditions such as kidney disease or diabetes, it may not be safe to follow a carnivorous diet.
- Not being mindful of the environmental impact: Meat consumption has been linked to environmental concerns such as deforestation, greenhouse gas emissions, and animal welfare. It is important to be mindful of the environmental impact of your dietary choices and choose high-quality, sustainably sourced animal-based foods whenever possible.
- Neglecting ethical considerations: While a carnivorous diet can offer numerous health benefits for some individuals, it is important to consider the ethical implications of

consuming animal-based foods. Choose high-quality, humanely raised animal-based foods whenever possible, and consider incorporating plant-based foods into your diet to support ethical and sustainable food choices.

In conclusion, while a carnivorous diet can offer numerous health benefits for some individuals, there are also common pitfalls to avoid when implementing this dietary pattern. By getting enough variety in your diet, monitoring your nutrient intake, being mindful of portion sizes, and considering the environmental and ethical implications of your dietary choices, you can safely and effectively implement a carnivorous diet that supports optimal health and well-being. As with any dietary pattern, it is important to consult with a healthcare professional and listen to your body to ensure that you are getting the right nutrition for your individual needs.

Addressing Concerns Around Nutrient Deficiencies And Health Risks

A carnivorous diet can provide numerous health benefits, but it is also important to address concerns around nutrient deficiencies and health risks. Here are some common concerns and strategies for addressing them:

Nutrient deficiencies:

One of the biggest concerns with a carnivorous diet is the potential for nutrient deficiencies. Plant-based foods are a major source of vitamins, minerals, and fiber, so it is important to make sure you are getting enough of these nutrients through animal-based foods. Some key nutrients to be mindful of include:

- Vitamin C: While meat contains some vitamin C, it may not be enough to meet daily needs. Consider incorporating small amounts of low-carbohydrate fruits such as berries or citrus fruits, or supplementing with a high-quality vitamin C supplement.
- Fiber: Animal-based foods tend to be low in fiber, which can lead to constipation and other digestive issues. Consider incorporating low-carbohydrate vegetables such as leafy greens, cruciferous vegetables, and other non-starchy vegetables into your diet to ensure that you are getting enough fiber.
- Calcium: While dairy products are a good source of calcium, it is still possible to get enough calcium from non-dairy sources such as bone-in fish or leafy green vegetables.
- Vitamin D: Vitamin D is important for bone health and immune function, and it can be difficult to get

enough from food alone. Consider getting regular sun exposure or supplementing with vitamin D to ensure that you are meeting your needs.

- Iron: Iron is important for red blood cell production and energy levels, and it can be found in high amounts in red meat, poultry, and organ meats. However, iron absorption can be inhibited by other components of meat, so it is important to get enough vitamin C and avoid consuming calcium-rich foods at the same time as iron-rich foods.

Health risks:

Another concern with a carnivorous diet is the potential for health risks such as heart disease, cancer, and kidney disease. While research on the long-term health effects of a carnivorous diet is limited, here are some strategies for mitigating these risks:

- Choose high-quality, nutrient-dense animal-based foods: Opt for grass-fed, pasture-raised, and wild-caught animal-based foods whenever possible, as these tend to be higher in nutrients and lower in harmful substances such as antibiotics and hormones.
- Avoid processed meats: Processed meats such as bacon, sausage, and deli meats have been linked to an increased risk of heart disease and cancer. Choose fresh, unprocessed meats instead.
- Monitor your fat intake: While fat is an important

      nutrient, it is possible to consume too much when following a carnivorous diet. Be mindful of your fat intake and choose leaner cuts of meat when possible.

- Monitor your blood markers: Get regular blood work to monitor your cholesterol levels, blood sugar levels, and other key markers of health. If you notice any concerning changes, consider adjusting your diet or working with a healthcare professional to develop a plan that meets your individual needs.

In conclusion, while a carnivorous diet can provide numerous health benefits, it is important to address concerns around nutrient deficiencies and health risks. By being mindful of your nutrient intake, choosing high-quality, nutrient-dense animal-based foods, avoiding processed meats, and monitoring your blood markers, you can safely and effectively implement a carnivorous diet that supports optimal health and well-being. As with any dietary pattern, it is important to consult with a healthcare professional and listen to your body to ensure that you are getting the right nutrition for your individual needs.

V. Conclusion

Final thoughts on the carnivorous diet and its potential benefits

In conclusion, the carnivorous diet is a dietary approach that involves consuming primarily animal-based foods while avoiding or minimizing plant-based foods. While this diet may seem restrictive, it has gained popularity in recent years due to its potential health benefits.

Some potential benefits of the carnivorous diet include weight loss, improved blood markers, increased energy, and better mental clarity. It may also help reduce inflammation and improve gut health, though more research is needed in these areas.

However, it is important to consider the potential risks and drawbacks of this diet as well. Nutrient deficiencies can be a concern, and there may be an increased risk of certain health conditions such as heart disease, cancer, and kidney disease.

The ethical and environmental implications of consuming a meat-based diet are also important to consider. Animal welfare, greenhouse gas emissions, and land use are all concerns when it comes to meat consumption, and choosing high-quality, sustainable sources of animal-based foods is important.

If you are considering a carnivorous diet, it is important to do your research and consult with a healthcare professional to ensure that you are meeting your nutrient needs and minimizing potential health risks. It may also be helpful to work with a registered dietitian or nutritionist to develop a meal plan that meets your individual needs.

In conclusion, the carnivorous diet is a controversial dietary approach that may have potential benefits for some individuals, but it is important to weigh the potential risks and drawbacks as well. If you choose to adopt this dietary pattern, be sure to do so in a mindful and informed way to ensure optimal health and well-being.

7 Days Meal Plan For Carnivorous Diet

Here is a sample 7-day meal plan for a carnivorous diet:

Day 1:

- Breakfast: Three fried eggs cooked in butter with two slices of bacon
- Lunch: Grilled chicken breast with a side of

steamed broccoli

- Dinner: Grilled steak with sautéed mushrooms and a side of spinach

Day 2:

- Breakfast: Omelette made with three eggs, cheddar cheese, and diced ham
- Lunch: Tuna salad with mayonnaise and chopped celery
- Dinner: Pork chops with roasted asparagus and a side of cauliflower mash

Day 3:

- Breakfast: Two lamb chops with a side of sliced avocado
- Lunch: Grilled shrimp with a side of zucchini noodles
- Dinner: Beef stir-fry with mixed vegetables and a side of sliced tomatoes

Day 4:

- Breakfast: Scrambled eggs cooked in butter with a side of bacon
- Lunch: Beef chili with sour cream and grated cheddar cheese
- Dinner: Grilled salmon with roasted Brussels sprouts and a side of sautéed spinach

Day 5:

- Breakfast: Two chicken sausages with a side of sliced avocado
- Lunch: Grilled chicken skewers with a side of

cucumber salad
- Dinner: Ribeye steak with sautéed onions and a side of roasted sweet potato
- Day 6:
- Breakfast: Three fried eggs cooked in bacon grease with a side of sliced tomato
- Lunch: Beef burger with lettuce, tomato, and mayonnaise
- Dinner: Roasted duck with a side of sautéed kale

Day 7:

- Breakfast: Grilled ham steak with a side of scrambled eggs
- Lunch: Tuna steak with a side of steamed green beans
- Dinner: Rack of lamb with a side of roasted mushrooms and a side salad

Note that this meal plan is just a sample and should be adjusted according to individual preferences and nutritional needs. It is important to consult with a healthcare professional before starting any new diet.

CHAPTER FIVE

Grilled Chicken Breast with Steamed Broccoli

Ingredients:

- 2 boneless, skinless chicken breasts
- Salt and black pepper, to taste
- 2 tablespoons olive oil
- 2 cups broccoli florets
- 1 tablespoon butter

Instructions:

- Preheat the grill to medium-high heat.
- Season the chicken breasts with salt, black pepper, and olive oil.
- Place the chicken breasts on the grill and cook for 6-8 minutes on each side, or until the internal temperature reaches 165°F.
- In a separate pot, bring 1 inch of water to a boil. Place the broccoli in a steamer basket and place the basket in the pot.
- Cover the pot with a lid and steam the broccoli for 5-7 minutes, or until it is tender but still has a bit of crunch.
- Remove the broccoli from the steamer basket and transfer to a serving dish.
- Melt the butter in a small saucepan and drizzle it

over the broccoli.

- Serve the grilled chicken breasts with the steamed broccoli on the side.

Grilled Steak with Sautéed Mushrooms and Spinach

Ingredients:

- 2 ribeye steaks
- Salt and black pepper, to taste
- 2 tablespoons olive oil
- 1 tablespoon butter
- 1 cup sliced mushrooms
- 2 cups fresh spinach leaves

Instructions:

- Preheat the grill to medium-high heat.
- Season the ribeye steaks with salt, black pepper, and olive oil.
- Place the steaks on the grill and cook for 4-6 minutes on each side, or until the internal temperature reaches your desired level of doneness.
- In a skillet over medium heat, melt the butter. Add the sliced mushrooms and sauté for 3-4 minutes, or until they are browned and tender.
- Add the fresh spinach leaves to the skillet and sauté for an additional 1-2 minutes, or until the spinach is wilted.
- Transfer the sautéed mushrooms and spinach to a serving dish.

- Serve the grilled ribeye steaks with the sautéed mushrooms and spinach on the side.

Omelette with Cheddar Cheese and Diced Ham

Ingredients:

- 3 eggs
- Salt and black pepper, to taste
- 1 tablespoon butter
- 1/4 cup shredded cheddar cheese
- 1/4 cup diced ham

Instructions:

- In a small bowl, beat the eggs with salt and black pepper.
- Melt the butter in a nonstick skillet over medium heat.
- Pour the beaten eggs into the skillet and tilt the pan to distribute the eggs evenly.
- As the eggs begin to set, use a spatula to lift the edges of the omelette and allow the uncooked eggs to flow underneath.
- Once the omelette is almost set, sprinkle the shredded cheddar cheese and diced ham over half of the omelette.
- Use the spatula to fold the other half of the omelette over the cheese and ham.
- Cook for an additional 1-2 minutes, or until the cheese is melted and the eggs are cooked through.
- Transfer the omelette to a serving dish and serve hot.

Grilled Salmon with Roasted Asparagus

Ingredients:

- 2 salmon fillets
- Salt and black pepper, to taste
- 2 tablespoons olive oil
- 1 pound asparagus spears, trimmed
- 1 tablespoon butter

Instructions:

- Preheat the grill to medium-high heat.
- Season the salmon fillets with salt, black pepper, and olive oil.
- PlacePlace the salmon fillets on the grill and cook for 4-6 minutes on each side, or until the internal temperature reaches 145°F.
- Preheat the oven to 425°F.
- Arrange the asparagus spears on a baking sheet and drizzle with olive oil. Season with salt and black pepper.
- Roast the asparagus in the oven for 12-15 minutes, or until it is tender and lightly browned.
- Melt the butter in a small saucepan and drizzle it over the roasted asparagus.
- Serve the grilled salmon fillets with the roasted asparagus on the side.

Pan-Seared Pork Chops with Creamed Spinach

Ingredients:

- 2 bone-in pork chops
- Salt and black pepper, to taste
- 2 tablespoons olive oil
- 1 tablespoon butter
- 1/2 cup heavy cream
- 2 cups fresh spinach leaves

Instructions:

- Season the pork chops with salt and black pepper.
- Heat the olive oil in a skillet over medium-high heat.
- Add the pork chops to the skillet and cook for 3-4 minutes on each side, or until the internal temperature reaches 145°F.
- Remove the pork chops from the skillet and let them rest for a few minutes before serving.
- In the same skillet, melt the butter over medium heat. Add the fresh spinach leaves and sauté for 2-3 minutes, or until the spinach is wilted.
- Add the heavy cream to the skillet and stir to combine.
- Continue cooking the creamed spinach until it is heated through and slightly thickened.
- Transfer the creamed spinach to a serving dish and serve hot, alongside the pan-seared pork chops.

Beef Stir-Fry with Broccoli and Bell Peppers

Ingredients:

- 1 pound flank steak, sliced into thin strips

- Salt and black pepper, to taste
- 2 tablespoons olive oil
- 1 tablespoon butter
- 2 cups broccoli florets
- 1 red bell pepper, sliced
- 1 green bell pepper, sliced
- 2 cloves garlic, minced
- 1/4 cup beef broth

Instructions:

- Season the flank steak strips with salt and black pepper.
- Heat the olive oil in a wok or large skillet over high heat.
- Add the beef strips to the wok and stir-fry for 2-3 minutes, or until browned on all sides. Remove the beef from the wok and set aside.
- Add the butter to the wok and melt over medium heat.
- Add the broccoli florets, bell peppers, and minced garlic to the wok and stir-fry for 3-4 minutes, or until the vegetables are slightly softened.
- Add the beef broth to the wok and stir to combine.
- Add the beef strips back to the wok and stir-fry for an additional 1-2 minutes, or until the beef is cooked through and the vegetables are tender-crisp.
- Transfer the beef stir-fry to a serving dish and serve hot.

Ribeye Steak with Grilled Asparagus

Ingredients:

- 1 ribeye steak
- 1 bunch of asparagus
- Salt
- Black pepper
- Olive oil

Instructions:

- Preheat grill or grill pan to high heat.
- Brush olive oil on both sides of the ribeye steak.
- Season the steak generously with salt and black pepper.
- Place the steak on the grill and cook for 4-5 minutes on each side for medium-rare or until desired doneness.
- While the steak is cooking, rinse the asparagus and trim the tough ends.
- Brush the asparagus with olive oil and season with salt and black pepper.
- Place the asparagus on the grill and cook for 2-3 minutes on each side or until tender.
- Serve the steak and asparagus hot.

Bacon and Eggs

Ingredients:

- 2 slices of bacon
- 2 large eggs
- Salt
- Black pepper
- Butter

Instructions:

- Heat a non-stick skillet over medium heat.
- Add the bacon slices and cook for 3-4 minutes on each side or until crispy.
- Remove the bacon from the skillet and set aside.
- Crack the eggs into the skillet and season with salt and black pepper.
- Cook the eggs for 2-3 minutes on each side or until the whites are set and the yolks are still runny.
- Remove the eggs from the skillet and serve with the bacon.

Pan-Seared Salmon with Roasted Brussels Sprouts

Ingredients:

- 1 salmon fillet
- 1 cup of Brussels sprouts
- Salt
- Black pepper
- Olive oil

Instructions:

- Preheat the oven to 400°F (200°C).
- Rinse the Brussels sprouts and cut off the stems.
- Toss the Brussels sprouts with olive oil and season with salt and black pepper.
- Spread the Brussels sprouts out on a baking sheet and roast in the oven for 20-25 minutes or until crispy and tender.

- Heat a non-stick skillet over medium-high heat.
- Brush olive oil on both sides of the salmon fillet and season with salt and black pepper.
- Place the salmon fillet in the skillet, skin side down.
- Cook the salmon for 4-5 minutes on the skin side or until the skin is crispy.
- Flip the salmon over and cook for an additional 2-3 minutes on the other side or until the fish is cooked through.
- Serve the salmon with the roasted Brussels sprouts.

Beef Burger with Bacon and Cheese

Ingredients:

- 1/2 lb ground beef
- 2 slices of bacon
- 1 slice of cheese
- Salt
- Black pepper
- Butter

Instructions:

- Preheat a non-stick skillet over medium-high heat.
- Form the ground beef into a patty and season with salt and black pepper.
- Melt a pat of butter in the skillet and add the beef patty.
- Cook the patty for 3-4 minutes on each side or

until it reaches your desired level of doneness.

- While the burger is cooking, fry the bacon in a separate skillet until crispy.
- Place the cooked burger patty on a plate and top with the slice of cheese and the bacon.
- Serve hot.

Grilled Chicken with Broccoli

Ingredients:

- 1 chicken breast
- 1 head of broccoli
- Salt
- Black pepper
- Olive oil

Instructions:

- Preheat grill or grill pan to high heat.
- Brush olive oil on both sides of the chicken breast and season with salt and black pepper.
- Place the chicken breast on the grill and cook for 6-8 minutes on each side or until the internal temperature reaches 165°F (75°C).
- While the chicken is cooking, rinse the broccoli and chop it into florets.
- Toss the broccoli florets with olive oil and season with salt and black pepper.
- Place the broccoli on the grill and cook for 2-3 minutes on each side or until tender and lightly charred.
- Serve the grilled chicken breast with the broccoli.

Tuna Salad

Ingredients:

- 1 can of tuna
- 2 tbsp mayonnaise
- 1 tbsp diced onion
- 1 tbsp diced celery
- Salt
- Black pepper

Instructions:

- Drain the can of tuna and transfer the tuna to a bowl.
- Add the mayonnaise, diced onion, and diced celery to the bowl and stir to combine.
- Season the tuna salad with salt and black pepper to taste.
- Serve the tuna salad on a bed of lettuce or with sliced vegetables on the side.

Ribeye Steak with Asparagus

Ingredients:

- 1 ribeye steak
- 1 bunch of asparagus
- Salt
- Black pepper
- Olive oil

Instructions:

- Preheat grill or grill pan to high heat.
- Brush olive oil on both sides of the ribeye steak and season with salt and black pepper.
- Place the steak on the grill and cook for 4-5 minutes on each side or until it reaches your desired level of doneness.
- While the steak is cooking, rinse the asparagus and snap off the woody ends.
- Toss the asparagus with olive oil and season with salt and black pepper.
- Place the asparagus on the grill and cook for 2-3 minutes on each side or until tender and lightly charred.
- Serve the ribeye steak with the asparagus.

Pork Chops with Brussels Sprouts

Ingredients:

- 2 pork chops
- 1 lb Brussels sprouts
- Salt
- Black pepper
- Olive oil

Instructions:

- Preheat oven to 400°F (200°C).
- Rinse the pork chops and pat dry with a paper towel. Season both sides with salt and black pepper.
- Heat a skillet over medium-high heat and add a drizzle of olive oil.

- Sear the pork chops on each side for 2-3 minutes until browned.
- Transfer the pork chops to a baking dish and bake for 10-15 minutes or until the internal temperature reaches 145°F (63°C).
- While the pork chops are cooking, rinse the Brussels sprouts and cut off the ends. Cut each Brussels sprout in half.
- Toss the Brussels sprouts with olive oil and season with salt and black pepper.
- Spread the Brussels sprouts in a single layer on a baking sheet and roast for 10-15 minutes or until tender and lightly browned.
- Serve the pork chops with the roasted Brussels sprouts.

Lamb Chops with Steamed Broccoli

Ingredients:

- 2 lamb chops
- 1 head of broccoli
- Salt
- Black pepper
- Butter

Instructions:

- Rinse the lamb chops and pat dry with a paper towel. Season both sides with salt and black pepper.
- Preheat a non-stick skillet over medium-high heat and add a pat of butter.

- Add the lamb chops to the skillet and cook for 3-4 minutes on each side or until it reaches your desired level of doneness.
- While the lamb chops are cooking, rinse the broccoli and chop it into florets.
- Fill a pot with 1-2 inches of water and place a steamer basket inside. Bring the water to a boil.
- Add the broccoli florets to the steamer basket and cover with a lid.
- Steam the broccoli for 3-4 minutes or until tender.
- Serve the lamb chops with the steamed broccoli.

CONCLUSION

In conclusion, the carnivorous diet has been a controversial topic in the world of nutrition and health, with strong opinions and arguments from both sides of the spectrum. While there are concerns around the ethical and environmental implications of consuming animal-based products, the research and anecdotal evidence suggest that the carnivorous diet can provide significant benefits for those who choose to follow it.

From weight loss and improved energy levels to better blood markers and mental clarity, the carnivorous diet has shown promise as a potential way to optimize health and well-being. However, it's important to note that this diet may not be suitable for everyone and can be challenging to sustain in the long term without careful planning and consideration.

Furthermore, it's essential to address concerns around potential nutrient deficiencies and health risks that may arise from following a carnivorous diet. With proper guidance and monitoring, it's possible to mitigate these risks and reap the benefits of a well-designed carnivorous diet.

Ultimately, whether or not to adopt a carnivorous diet is a personal choice that requires careful consideration of individual values, health goals, and dietary preferences. The key is to stay informed and work with qualified health professionals to develop a personalized plan that supports optimal health and well-being.

www.ingramcontent.com/pod-product-compliance
Lightning Source LLC
Chambersburg PA
CBHW050701250726

48662CB00002B/784